My Favorite Juice Recipes Book

A record of the best juice recipes that I have found or created so far

Journal Easy

© 2014

www.journaleasy.com – making journal writing effortless

Juice Name:

Ingredients:

Comments:

Juice Name:

Ingredients:

Comments:

Juice Name:

Ingredients:

Comments:

Juice Name:

Ingredients:

Comments:

Juice Name:

Ingredients:

Comments:

Juice Name:

Ingredients:

Comments:

Juice Name:

Ingredients:

Comments:

Juice Name:

Ingredients:

Comments:

Juice Name:

Ingredients:

Comments:

Juice Name:

Ingredients:

Comments:

Juice Name:

Ingredients:

Comments:

Juice Name:

Ingredients:

Comments:

Juice Name:

Ingredients:

Comments:

Juice Name:

Ingredients:

Comments:

Juice Name:

Ingredients:

Comments:

Juice Name:

Ingredients:

Comments:

Juice Name:

Ingredients:

Comments:

Juice Name:

Ingredients:

Comments:

Juice Name:

Ingredients:

Comments:

Juice Name:

Ingredients:

Comments:

Juice Name:

Ingredients:

Comments:

Juice Name:

Ingredients:

Comments:

Juice Name:

Ingredients:

Comments:

Juice Name:

Ingredients:

Comments:

Juice Name:

Ingredients:

Comments:

Juice Name:

Ingredients:

Comments:

Juice Name:

Ingredients:

Comments:

Juice Name:

Ingredients:

Comments:

Juice Name:

Ingredients:

Comments:

Juice Name:

Ingredients:

Comments:

Juice Name:

Ingredients:

Comments:

Juice Name:

Ingredients:

Comments:

Juice Name:

Ingredients:

Comments:

Juice Name:

Ingredients:

Comments:

Juice Name:

Ingredients:

Comments:

Juice Name:

Ingredients:

Comments:

Juice Name:

Ingredients:

Comments:

Juice Name:

Ingredients:

Comments:

Juice Name:

Ingredients:

Comments:

Juice Name:

Ingredients:

Comments:

Juice Name:

Ingredients:

Comments:

Juice Name:

Ingredients:

Comments:

Juice Name:

Ingredients:

Comments:

Juice Name:

Ingredients:

Comments:

Juice Name:

Ingredients:

Comments:

Juice Name:

Ingredients:

Comments:

Juice Name:

Ingredients:

Comments:

Juice Name:

Ingredients:

Comments:

Juice Name:

Ingredients:

Comments:

Juice Name:

Ingredients:

Comments:

Juice Name:

Ingredients:

Comments:

Juice Name:

Ingredients:

Comments:

Juice Name:

Ingredients:

Comments:

Juice Name:

Ingredients:

Comments:

Juice Name:

Ingredients:

Comments:

Juice Name:

Ingredients:

Comments:

Juice Name:

Ingredients:

Comments:

Juice Name:

Ingredients:

Comments:

Juice Name:

Ingredients:

Comments:

Juice Name:

Ingredients:

Comments:

Juice Name:

Ingredients:

Comments:

Juice Name:

Ingredients:

Comments:

Juice Name:

Ingredients:

Comments:

Juice Name:

Ingredients:

Comments:

Juice Name:

Ingredients:

Comments:

Juice Name:

Ingredients:

Comments:

Juice Name:

Ingredients:

Comments:

Juice Name:

Ingredients:

Comments:

Juice Name:

Ingredients:

Comments:

Juice Name:

Ingredients:

Comments:

Juice Name:

Ingredients:

Comments:

Juice Name:

Ingredients:

Comments:

Juice Name:

Ingredients:

Comments:

Juice Name:

Ingredients:

Comments:

Juice Name:

Ingredients:

Comments:

Juice Name:

Ingredients:

Comments:

Juice Name:

Ingredients:

Comments:

Juice Name:

Ingredients:

Comments:

Juice Name:

Ingredients:

Comments:

Juice Name:

Ingredients:

Comments:

Juice Name:

Ingredients:

Comments:

Juice Name:

Ingredients:

Comments:

Juice Name:

Ingredients:

Comments:

Juice Name:

Ingredients:

Comments:

Juice Name:

Ingredients:

Comments:

Juice Name:

Ingredients:

Comments:

Juice Name:

Ingredients:

Comments:

Juice Name:

Ingredients:

Comments:

Juice Name:

Ingredients:

Comments:

Juice Name:

Ingredients:

Comments:

Juice Name:

Ingredients:

Comments:

Juice Name:

Ingredients:

Comments:

Juice Name:

Ingredients:

Comments:

Juice Name:

Ingredients:

Comments:

Juice Name:

Ingredients:

Comments:

Juice Name:

Ingredients:

Comments:

Juice Name:

Ingredients:

Comments:

Juice Name:

Ingredients:

Comments:

Juice Name:

Ingredients:

Comments:

Juice Name:

Ingredients:

Comments:

Juice Name:

Ingredients:

Comments:

Juice Name:

Ingredients:

Comments:

Juice Name:

Ingredients:

Comments:

Juice Name:

Ingredients:

Comments:

Juice Name:

Ingredients:

Comments:

Juice Name:

Ingredients:

Comments:

Juice Name:

Ingredients:

Comments:

Juice Name:

Ingredients:

Comments:

Juice Name:

Ingredients:

Comments:

Juice Name:

Ingredients:

Comments:

Juice Name:

Ingredients:

Comments:

Juice Name:

Ingredients:

Comments:

Juice Name:

Ingredients:

Comments:

Juice Name:

Ingredients:

Comments:

Juice Name:

Ingredients:

Comments:

Juice Name:

Ingredients:

Comments:

Juice Name:

Ingredients:

Comments:

Juice Name:

Ingredients:

Comments:

Juice Name:

Ingredients:

Comments:

Juice Name:

Ingredients:

Comments:

Juice Name:

Ingredients:

Comments:

Juice Name:

Ingredients:

Comments:

Juice Name:

Ingredients:

Comments:

Juice Name:

Ingredients:

Comments:

Juice Name:

Ingredients:

Comments:

Juice Name:

Ingredients:

Comments:

Juice Name:

Ingredients:

Comments:

Juice Name:

Ingredients:

Comments:

Juice Name:

Ingredients:

Comments:

Juice Name:

Ingredients:

Comments:

Juice Name:

Ingredients:

Comments:

Juice Name:

Ingredients:

Comments:

Juice Name:

Ingredients:

Comments:

Juice Name:

Ingredients:

Comments:

Juice Name:

Ingredients:

Comments:

Juice Name:

Ingredients:

Comments:

Juice Name:

Ingredients:

Comments:

Juice Name:

Ingredients:

Comments:

Juice Name:

Ingredients:

Comments:

Juice Name:

Ingredients:

Comments:

Juice Name:

Ingredients:

Comments:

Juice Name:

Ingredients:

Comments:

Juice Name:

Ingredients:

Comments:

Juice Name:

Ingredients:

Comments:

Juice Name:

Ingredients:

Comments:

Juice Name:

Ingredients:

Comments:

Juice Name:

Ingredients:

Comments:

Juice Name:

Ingredients:

Comments:

Juice Name:

Ingredients:

Comments:

Juice Name:

Ingredients:

Comments:

My Favorite Juice Books & Resources

If you don't have a great juicer yet, go to: www.vitalityjuicers.com in the USA & Canada or www.vitalityjuicers.co.uk in the UK. These sites research & find the best juicers & blenders that can be bought online.

My Favorite Juice Books & Resources

www.journaleasy.com – making journal writing effortless

My Favorite Juice Books & Resources

My Favorite Juice Books & Resources

www.ingramcontent.com/pod-product-compliance
Lightning Source LLC
LaVergne TN
LVHW011710060526
838200LV00051B/2847